# richar[d]

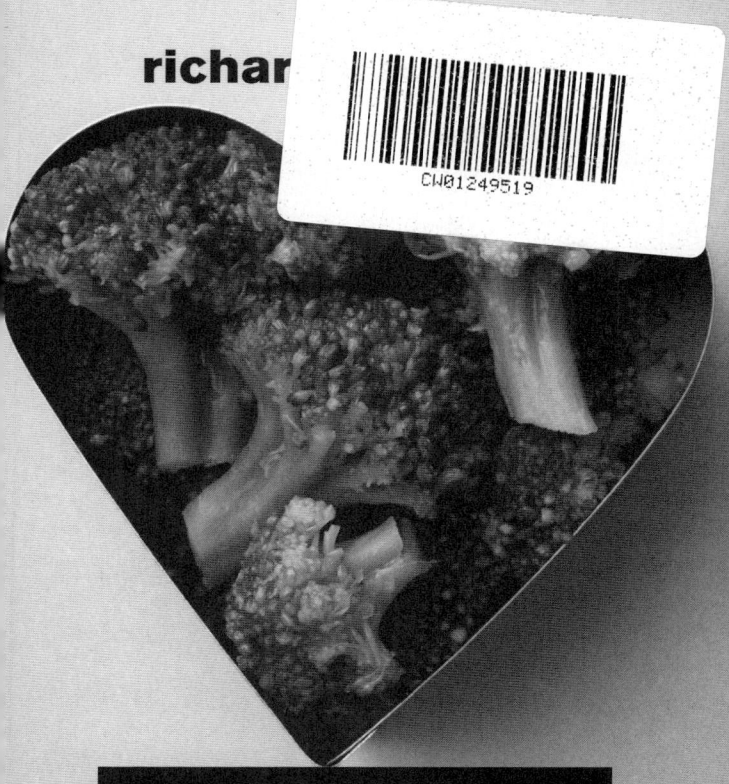

# HOW TO POSTPONE YOUR HEART ATTACK

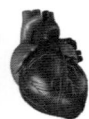

First published 2009

Copyright © 2009

All rights reserved. No part of this publication may be reproduced in any form without prior permission from the publisher.

British Library Cataloguing in Publication Data. A catalogue record for this book is available from the British Library.

ISBN 978-1-906381-61-5

Published by Autumn House, Grantham, Lincolnshire.
Printed in Thailand.

Unless otherwise indicated, Bible verses have been taken
from the *King James Version* of the Bible.
Other versions used, indicated by initials:
*New International Version* (Hodder and Stoughton) = NIV
*The Message* (NavPress) = MGE

### On the beat!

This little **heart-to-heart** will help you to recognise the risk factors for your heart attack (properly called 'cardiac arrest'), and so postpone the event *indefinitely*. You don't want to leave your heart in San Francisco, or anywhere else for that matter, when with appropriate care it will look after you.

When I was one-and-twenty
I heard a wise man say,
'Give crowns and pounds and guineas
But not your heart away!'
*A. E. Housman (1859-1936)*

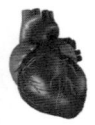

*Keep thy heart with all diligence; for out of it are the issues of life.*
Proverbs 4:23

# Health is...
A state of total physical, mental and social well-being, not merely the absence of disease.
*World Health Organisation*

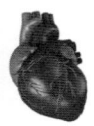

## Health is . . .
Physical soundness,
mental soundness,
spiritual soundness.
*Concise Oxford Dictionary*

It is highly dishonourable for a reasonable soul to live in so divinely built a mansion as the body she resides in, altogether unacquainted with the exquisite structure of it.
*Robert Boyle (1627-1691)*

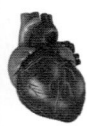

# Normal heart

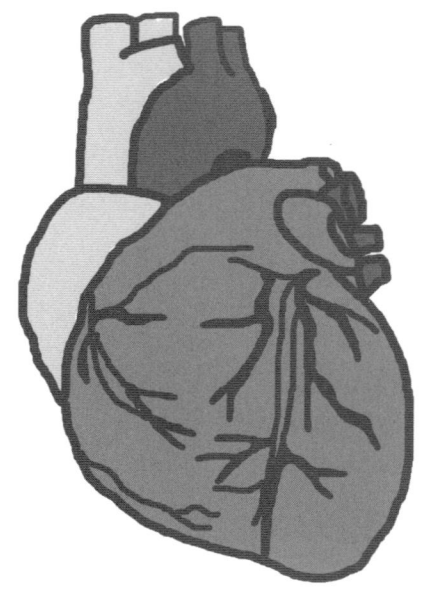

# Heart showing coronary arteries

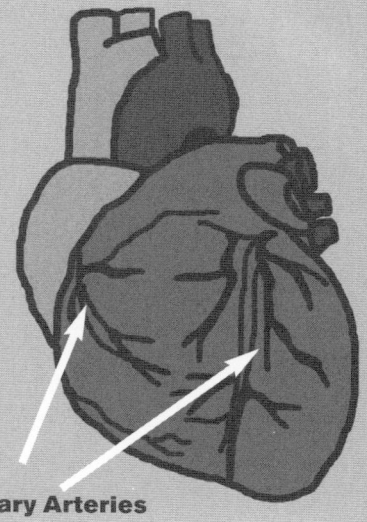

**Coronary Arteries**

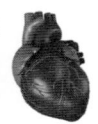

## Heart damaged by a clot in a coronary artery

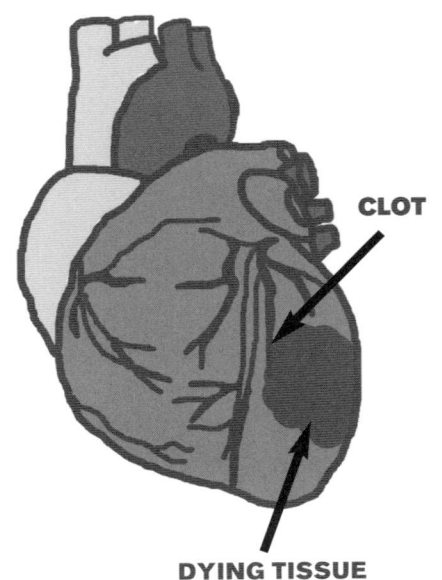

CLOT

DYING TISSUE

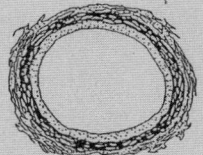
Normal artery

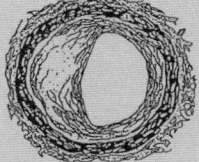
Partially obstructed artery

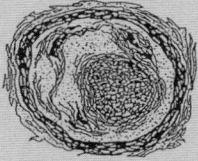
Completely obstructed artery

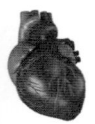

- Your heart weighs 8-10 ounces.
- It beats 50-100 times a minute, 100,000 times a day for as long as you live.

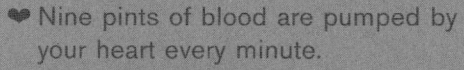

- Nine pints of blood are pumped by your heart every minute.
- Around 60,000 miles of arteries, veins and capillaries carry your blood.

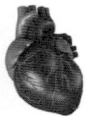

> But the beating of my own heart
> Was all the sound I heard.
> *R. Monckton Milnes (1809-1885)*

- For coronary thrombosis and heart-rate disorders, every minute that passes untreated means a 10% less chance of survival.
- If you are four minutes without resuscitation following a coronary event, your brain is starved of blood and could suffer irreversible damage.

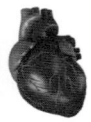

# Primary risk factors for heart disease
- ❤ Obesity
- ❤ Cigarette smoking
- ❤ Hypertension
- ❤ High blood cholesterol

*Framingham Study (1948-present)*

## Obesity
♥ Being overweight will increase the risk.

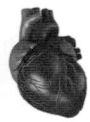

## Cigarette smoking
- ❤ The more cigarettes smoked, the greater the risk.
- ❤ The risk of heart attack or angina pectoris is increased about 70% in smokers.
- ❤ Smoking constricts the blood vessels of the heart and increases blood pressure.

# Blood pressure
- ♥ The higher the blood pressure, the greater the risk.
- ♥ The greatest pressure (systolic) required to close the flow of blood from the heart to the brachial artery, measured against the pressure (diastolic) in the resting artery.

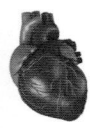

Chronic high blood pressure accelerates the disease process in the coronary arteries and places undue strain on the heart muscle itself, making it thicken and eventually lose its flexibility and ability to function adequately. Heart failure follows.
*Dr Peter N. Landless*

## High blood pressure

may cause:
- ❤ Headaches
- ❤ Breathlessness
- ❤ Dizziness
- ❤ Disturbed vision
- ❤ Most frequently – no symptoms (blood pressure is a silent killer)

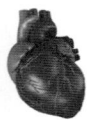

# Blood pressure ranges

|  | *Diastolic* | *Systolic* |
| --- | --- | --- |
| Very high | 110+ | 180+ |
| Moderately high | 100-110 | 160-180 |
| Slightly high | 90-100 | 140-160 |
| Optimum | 80 or less | 120 or less |

## Children, exercise and blood pressure

Children who are physically fit have lower blood pressure than their sedentary counterparts.
*T. F. Kirn, JAMA*

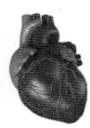

## Aerobics and blood pressure

In a study of African-American adolescent girls . . . it was found that the aerobic exercise group had a greater decrease in systolic blood pressure than the group receiving standard physical education.
*C. K. Ewart et al, AJPH.*

## Blood cholesterol
♥ The higher the cholesterol, the greater the risk.

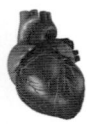

## Factors influencing blood cholesterol

- Liver converts saturated fat to cholesterol.
- Cholesterol is also absorbed directly from food.
- Obesity, genetics, and other dietary factors influence the amount.

# The contrasting actions of HDL and LDL cholesterol

**High Density Lipoprotein (HDL)**
Removes fatty substance from artery wall.

High levels of HDL associated with low levels of CHD.

**Low Density Lipoprotein (LDL)**
Promotes deposition of fatty substance in artery wall.

High levels of LDL associated with high rates of CHD.

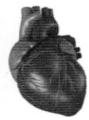

# Cholesterol levels

|  | *Cholesterol* | *LDL* | *HDL* |
|---|---|---|---|
| High-risk | 2.4g/l+ | 1.6g/l+ | less than 0.35g/l |
| At risk | 2-2.4 g/l | 1.3-1.6g/l | – |
| Ideal | less than 2g/l | less than 1.3g/l | 0.4-0.55g/l |

Elevated cholesterol levels are very important in the genesis of atherosclerosis, but they are not synonymous with the disease. Many genetic factors and environmental risk factors can increase or decrease the tolerance to elevated cholesterol levels.
*Dr Alexander Leaf, Harvard Medical School.*

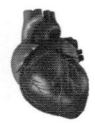

In societies in which the mean cholesterol levels are 150 or lower without the use of drugs, coronary heart disease is essentially unknown as a public health problem.
*Dr Alexander Leaf, Harvard Medical School*

Vegetarians have low levels of total cholesterol, very low LDL levels, and very low rates of coronary heart disease even though their HDL levels tend to be low and their triglyceride levels tend to be high.
*Dr Dean Ornish*

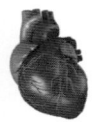

Even a single meal that is high in fat and cholesterol may cause your arteries to constrict and your blood to clot more quickly due to the release of hormones such as Factor VII and thromboxane. Emotional stress may cause your arteries to constrict (via the sympathetic nervous system) and your blood to clot more quickly (via stress hormones like adrenaline and noradrenaline). Nicotine may cause your arteries to constrict and your blood to clot more quickly.
*Dr Dean Ornish*

- Triglycerides are glycerine and three fatty molecules that have bonded for transportation around the body via the liver. They constitute the usual form of fat found in the blood.
- If the diet is rich in calories, carbohydrates and cholesterol, their level is raised and they contribute to disorders such as atherosclerosis and coronary heart disease.

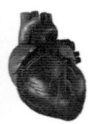

## Dietary factors:
- ♥ The more cholesterol and saturated fat, the higher the blood cholesterol level and blood pressure.
- ♥ High blood cholesterol levels and high blood pressure increase the coronary heart disease risk.
- ♥ The more cholesterol and saturated fat, the greater the coronary heart disease risk, *even if blood cholesterol levels and blood pressure do not rise by much.*

- People eating low-fat, low-cholesterol vegetarian diets have low blood pressure and low blood cholesterol levels in childhood which remain low as they age, and have low heart disease risk.
- People eating a typical US/UK diet have low blood pressure and low blood cholesterol levels in childhood which increase as they age, and have high heart disease risk.

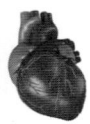

# Secondary risk factors for heart disease
- ❤ Physical inactivity
- ❤ Low HDL cholesterol levels
- ❤ Diabetes
- ❤ Stress
- ❤ Alcohol intake
- ❤ Oestrogen use

*Framingham Study (1948-present)*

## Physical inactivity
- ♥ The less exercise taken, the greater the risk.
- ♥ Only 2% of our society gets enough physical activity in their routine occupations to stay physically fit.

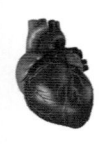

I believe every human has a finite number of heartbeats. I don't intend to waste any of mine running around doing exercises.
*Neil Armstrong*

## 'Apple' vs 'pear' shape body

♥ Apple shape increases risk of heart disease, diabetes or cancer.
♥ Waist in
(f) more than 35 inches/89.5cms;
(m) more than 40 inches/102cms.

## Apples 'n' pears

Fat that accumulates around your waist seems to be more biologically active as it secretes inflammatory proteins that contribute to atherosclerotic plaque build-up, whereas fat around your hips doesn't appear to increase risk for cardiovascular disease at all.
*Professor James de Lemnos, J. Am. Coll. Cardiology*

## Low HDL cholesterol levels

♥ Having low amounts of the protective HDL cholesterol can be as harmful as having high levels of the damaging LDL cholesterol.

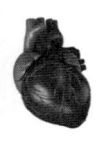

## Diabetes
- People with diabetes have a 4-7 times higher risk of coronary heart disease.
- The blood vessels of the heart are damaged by excess blood sugar, they lose their elasticity and attract plaque deposits.

## Stress

- ♥ Stress, in most people, will increase the risk of heart disease.
- ♥ Stresses may be due to role or status in a community, work, home, or relationships in general posing a regular and consistent threat to health with the heart as a 'target organ'.

## A survey of 99,029 Italian railway workers found:

The combination of high job responsibility and low level of physical work was associated with an increased risk of heart attack.

Men with the most anger and hostility have the highest risk of heart disease.

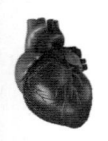

Men who had low control over the demands of their jobs were 1.8 times more likely to die from heart disease than men with more control were; men who experienced a low level of social support from co-workers were 2.6 times more vulnerable to cardiovascular death.

The tighter the constraints within which a family must operate, the fewer the demands which can be satisfied, and the more people's interests conflict. The smaller the resources, the less the capacity to overcome unforeseen difficulties, accidents, breakages or losses. The greater the potential sources of stress and conflict, the more family life and social support will suffer.
*Richard G. Wilkinson*

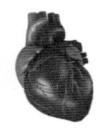

The strongest predictor of longevity was work satisfaction. The second best predictor was overall 'happiness'. . . . Other factors are undoubtedly important – diet, exercise, medical care, and genetic inheritance. But research findings suggest that these factors may account for only about 25% of the risk factors in heart disease, the major cause of death. That is, if cholesterol, blood pressure, smoking, glucose level, serum uric acid, and so forth, were perfectly controlled, only about one fourth of coronary heart disease could be controlled . . . it appears that work role, work conditions and other social factors may contribute heavily to this 'unexplained' 75% of risk factors.
*Vincente Navarro*

# Dartmouth Medical School researchers reported that:

Older people who underwent open-heart surgery for either coronary artery or aortic valve disease – and who lacked social support from an organised group or said they received no comfort from religion – were three times more likely to die within six months of the operation than those who said they got solace from community groups or religion.

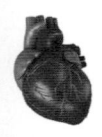

## Alcohol intake

- Alcohol adversely affects the functions of the heart muscle and contributes to chronic disease of the heart muscle which eventually leads to heart failure.

Monday peak in deaths from coronary heart disease in Scotland may be partly attributable to increased drinking at the weekend, although other mechanisms, such as work-related stress, may be important.

The possible link between binge drinking and deaths from coronary heart disease has potentially important public health implications and merits further investigation.
*C. Evans et al, BMJ*

## The regional heart study

- Preliminary data from the UK regions appeared to show that abstainers were at greater risk of heart disease than moderate drinkers.
- The media and now urban myth took the U-shaped graph to mean that 'a little alcohol is good for the heart'.

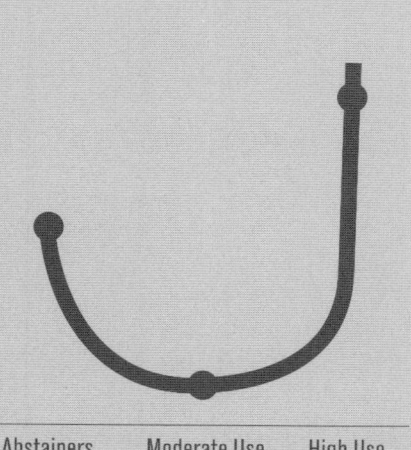

# The U-shaped curve

| | | | |
|---|---|---|---|
| High | | | ● |
| Medium | ● | | |
| Low | | | |
| | Abstainers | Moderate Use | High Use |

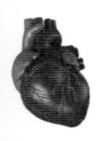

- It was later discovered that the 'abstainers' in the data were largely people who had been told to quit drinking *because* they had heart disease *(sick quitters)*.
- It is speculated that if the research were to be reported using lifelong total abstainers, the result would most likely be a J-shaped graph.

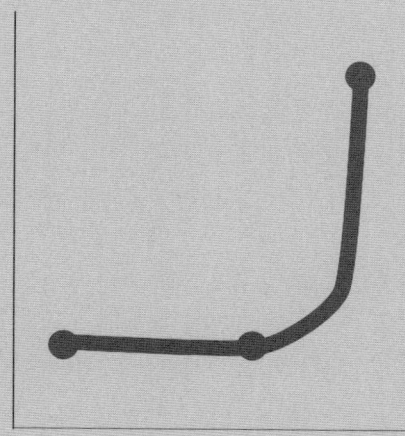

# The J-shaped curve

| | |
|---|---|
| High | |
| Medium | |
| Low | |
| | Abstainers　　Moderate Use　　High Use |

## Alcohol and the heart

Results from a Scottish study showed that:

... there was no relation between mortality from coronary heart disease and alcohol consumption once adjustments were made for potential confounding factors.

*Professor G. D. Smith et al, BMJ*

## Oestrogen use
♥ Oestrogen use increases the risk of abnormal blood clotting so should not be used by people with a family history of heart conditions or in those about to undergo surgery. The use of oestrogen drugs may increase a hypertension risk.

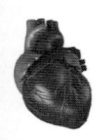

- Smoking tobacco while using oestrogen drugs significantly increases the risk of abnormal clotting of the blood, resulting in cardiac arrest, stroke or pulmonary embolism.

# Other contributing factors
- Family history.
- Personality type.
- Water hardness or softness.
- Multiplication of symptoms.

## Family history

- The longer the parents live, the less risk for their children.

## Personality type
- The type A personality will be at greater risk of coronary heart disease.

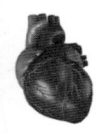

## Measuring type A behaviour

Circle one number for each of the statements below which best reflects the way you behave in your everyday life. For example, if you are generally on time for appointments. For the first point you would circle a number between 7 and 11. If you are usually casual about appointments, you would circle one of the lower numbers between 1 and 5.

## Scoring

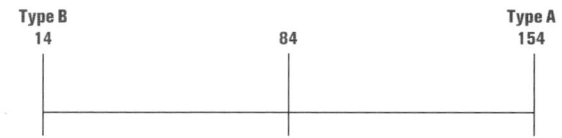

| Type B | | Type A |
|:---|:---:|---:|
| 14 | 84 | 154 |

*Source: Cooper's adaptation of the Bortner Type A Scale*

The higher the score received on this questionnaire, the more firmly an individual can be classified as type A. For example, 154 points is the highest score and indicates the maximum type A coronary prone personality. It is important to understand that there are no distinct divisions between type A and type B. Rather, people fall somewhere on a continuum leaning more towards one type than the other. Eighty-four is the average score. Anyone with a score above that is inclined towards type A behaviour.

| | | |
|---|---|---|
| Casual about appointments | 1 2 3 4 5 6 7 8 9 10 11 | Never late |
| Not competitive | 1 2 3 4 5 6 7 8 9 10 11 | Very competitive |
| Good listener | 1 2 3 4 5 6 7 8 9 10 11 | Anticipates what others are going to say (nods, attempts to finish for them) |
| Never feels rushed (even under pressure) | 1 2 3 4 5 6 7 8 9 10 11 | Always rushed |
| Can wait patiently | 1 2 3 4 5 6 7 8 9 10 11 | Impatient while waiting |
| Takes things one at a time | 1 2 3 4 5 6 7 8 9 10 11 | Tries to do many things at once, thinks about what will do next |
| Slow, deliberate talker | 1 2 3 4 5 6 7 8 9 10 11 | Emphatic in speech, fast and forceful |
| Cares about satisfying him/herself no matter what others may think | 1 2 3 4 5 6 7 8 9 10 11 | Wants good job recognised by others |
| Slow doing things | 1 2 3 4 5 6 7 8 9 10 11 | Fast (eating, walking) |
| Easy-going | 1 2 3 4 5 6 7 8 9 10 11 | Hard driving (pushing self and others) |
| Expresses feelings | 1 2 3 4 5 6 7 8 9 10 11 | Hides feelings |
| Many outside interests | 1 2 3 4 5 6 7 8 9 10 11 | Few interests outside work/home |
| Unambitious | 1 2 3 4 5 6 7 8 9 10 11 | Ambitious |
| Casual | 1 2 3 4 5 6 7 8 9 10 11 | Eager to get things done |

## Water hardness
- The softer the tap water, the greater the risk.
- The incidence of coronary heart disease in towns with a very soft water supply is about 40% greater than in towns with very hard water.

## Multiplication of symptoms

- ♥ If you have high blood pressure, you're three times more likely to have a stroke.
- ♥ If you smoke, you're twice as likely to have a stroke.
- ♥ If you do not exercise regularly, you're twice as likely to have a stroke.
- ♥ If all three apply to you, *you're twelve times more likely* to have a stroke, because risk factors multiply up.

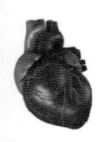

# The Alameda County (California) Study

Set up in 1959 to:

- Assess the level of health (physical, mental and social) of persons living in Alameda County, CA, ... and ... to study the influence of certain ways of living, specifically, common health practices and social relationships on physical health status.
- The research showed that practising one or a combination of health habits resulted in lower mortality rates from heart disease over a nine-year period across a range of common health habits as presented in the following pages.

## People with the best heart health were those who:

- ❤ Never smoked.
- ❤ Drank less than four alcoholic drinks a week.
- ❤ Had breakfast every day.
- ❤ Rarely ate between meals.
- ❤ Slept 7-8 hours a night.
- ❤ Often engaged in exercise.
- ❤ Were less than 10% overweight (men less than 20%).

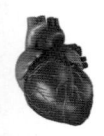

## Health habits

(% dead in 9 years – women)

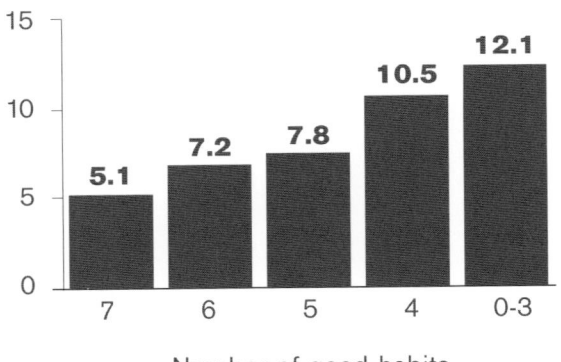

| Number of good habits | % dead |
|---|---|
| 7 | 5.1 |
| 6 | 7.2 |
| 5 | 7.8 |
| 4 | 10.5 |
| 0-3 | 12.1 |

## Health habits
(% dead in 9 years – men)

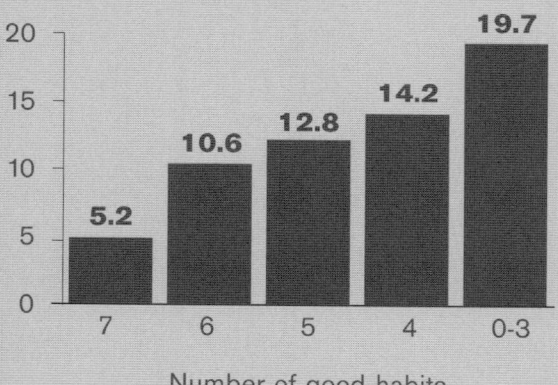

| Number of good habits | % dead in 9 years |
|---|---|
| 7 | 5.2 |
| 6 | 10.6 |
| 5 | 12.8 |
| 4 | 14.2 |
| 0-3 | 19.7 |

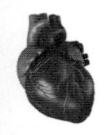

## Breakfast
(% dead in 9 years)

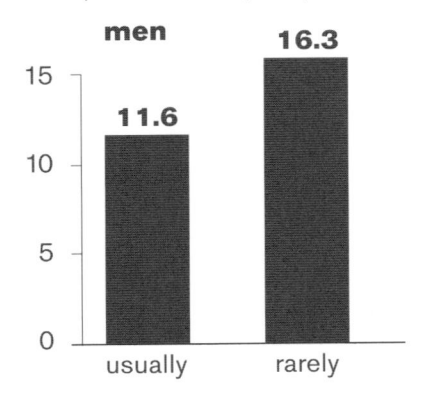

**men**

| | usually | rarely |
|---|---|---|
| | 11.6 | 16.3 |

# Breakfast
(% dead in 9 years)

**women**

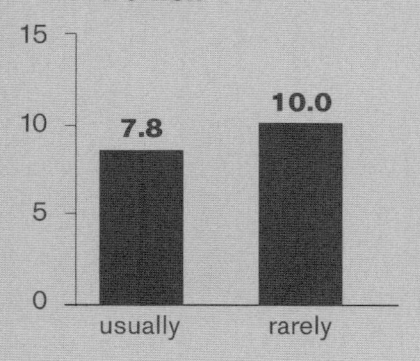

| | usually | rarely |
|---|---|---|
| | 7.8 | 10.0 |

## Sleep

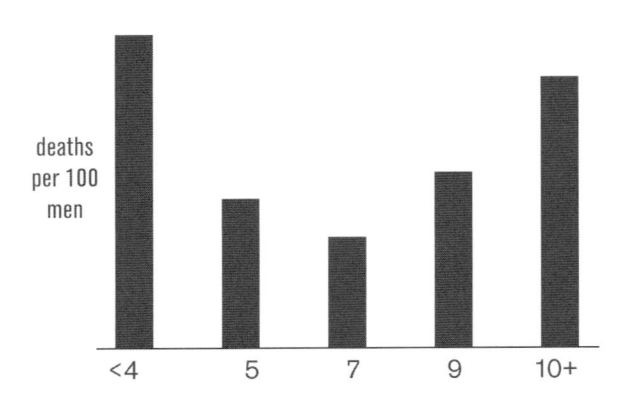

deaths per 100 men

<4    5    7    9    10+

ill health ——— optimum hours of sleep ——— ill health

# Exercise
(% dead in 9 years – men)

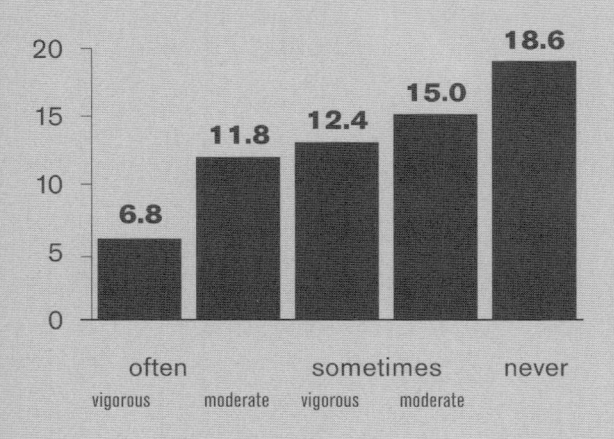

| often | | sometimes | | never |
|---|---|---|---|---|
| vigorous | moderate | vigorous | moderate | |
| 6.8 | 11.8 | 12.4 | 15.0 | 18.6 |

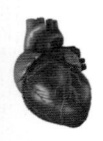

- *A merry heart maketh a cheerful countenance....* Proverbs 15:13
- *A merry heart doeth good like a medicine....* Proverbs 17:22
- *... a light heart lives long.*
  *William Shakespeare*

## Happiness
(% dead in 9 years - men)

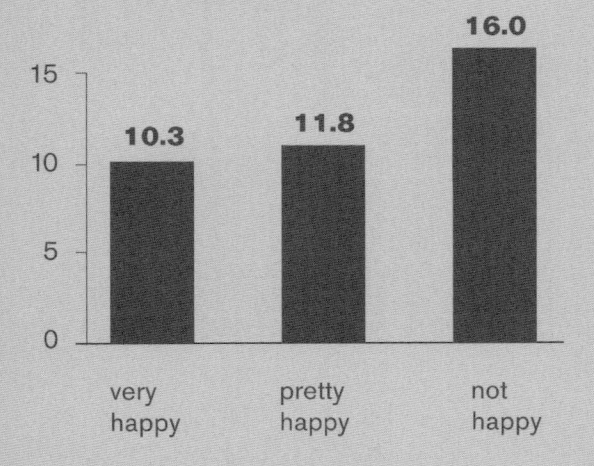

| Category | % dead |
|---|---|
| very happy | 10.3 |
| pretty happy | 11.8 |
| not happy | 16.0 |

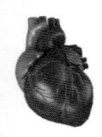

## Happiness

(% dead in 9 years – women)

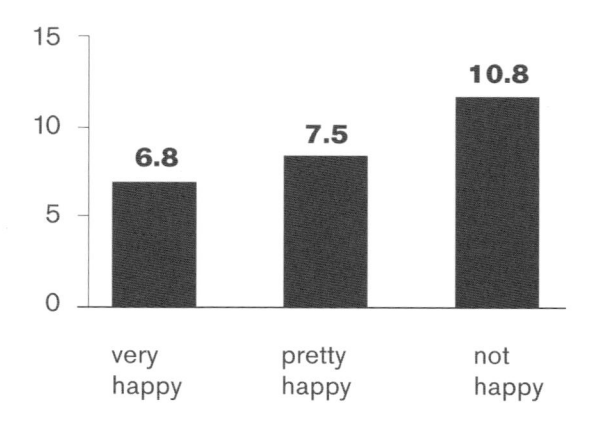

- very happy: 6.8
- pretty happy: 7.5
- not happy: 10.8

# Role of stress in ischemic heart disease across the age range

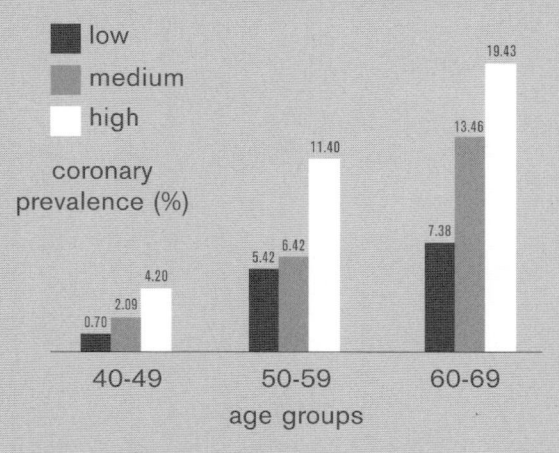

- ■ low
- ■ medium
- □ high

coronary prevalence (%)

| age group | low | medium | high |
|---|---|---|---|
| 40-49 | 0.70 | 2.09 | 4.20 |
| 50-59 | 5.42 | 6.42 | 11.40 |
| 60-69 | 7.38 | 13.46 | 19.43 |

age groups

H. I. & L. G. Russek

## Stages of heart disease
- **Wrong habits** — violation of laws of life
- **Indicator** — high cholesterol
- **Body changes** — hardened arteries
- **Sign of disease** — abnormal ECG
- **Symptoms** — pain
- **Attack** — heart attack
- **Death**

# Heart attack pathway

**CONTRIBUTING FACTORS**
- Smoking
- Unfitness
- Fatness
- Sugar
- Fat

↓

**MAIN EFFECTS OF LIFE FACTORS**

↓

**SUBSIDIARY OUTCOMES**
- Raised BP
- Blood clots
- Premature ageing

- Stress hormones released
- Fat (without outlet) freed to fuel muscles
- Raised cholesterol and triglycerides

➤ HEART ATTACK

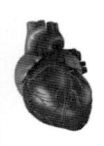

## Exercise pulse rate

180 minus your age

Exercise at a heart rate no greater than 180 minus your age. (This gives you a target rate between 75% and 80% of your maximum.)

# Get your heart working for you

72 x 60 x 24 = 103,680 beats per day

If by exercising 1 hour a day your heart rate drops to 60 beats/min

1 x 60 x 140 (for the hour you exercise) = 8,400
23 x 60 (min/hr) x 60 (new pulse rate) = 82,800

Total for the 24 hours at the new rate =
82,800 + 8,400 = 91,200

103,680 - 91,200 = 12,480: more than a 10% saving

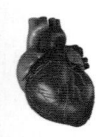

## The 3-minute Kasch Pulse Recovery Step Test

*Equipment:*
- ♥ A solid bench 12 inches high or step.
- ♥ A stop watch or clock with sweep second hand.

*Procedure:*
- ♥ Do not eat for two hours prior to test, or smoke for one hour prior to test. ♥ Rest five minutes prior to test. ♥ Begin stepping with stronger leg, bringing other foot up beside lead off foot with full extension of body. Continue for one minute. Without missing a step lead off with weaker leg for second minute, then return to stronger leg for third minute. Duration three minutes. ♥ Step up 24 per minute or two steps per five seconds. ♥ Stop and sit.
- ♥ Begin counting pulse immediately upon sitting. Count for one minute and classify according to table opposite.

# Standards, Kasch Pulse Recovery Test

| Classification | 0-1 min PR after exercise |
|---|---|
| Excellent | 71-78 |
| Very good | 79-83 |
| Average | 84-99 |
| Below average | 100-107 |
| Poor | 108-118 |

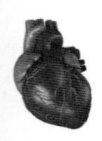

## Ten tips for postponing your heart attack

1. Know and keep to your ideal weight.

2. Choose complex carbohydrates (wholemeal, wholegrain items) but avoid overeating (notwithstanding the Anglo-French heart health paradox).

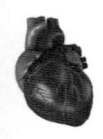

## Anglo-French heart health

... the difference is due to the time lag between increases in consumption of animal fat and serum cholesterol concentrations and the resulting increase in mortality from heart disease similar to the recognised time lag between smoking and lung cancer. Consumption of animal fat and serum cholesterol concentrations increased only recently in France but did so decades ago in Britain.
*Law & Wald, BMJ*

# 3. Take plenty of fruits and vegetables.

# Dietary recommendations for heart disease

*Increase:*
Vegetarian food
Complex carbohydrates/fibre
Grain, vegetables, fruit

## Dietary recommendations for heart disease

*Lower:*
Total fat
Saturated fat/meat
Calories (to match ideal weight)
Refined sugar
Alcohol
Salt

Long-term vegetarians
had the lowest risk of CHD
of any identifiable group,
much lower than marathon
runners. . . .
*Dr Dean Ornish*

4. Use rape or olive oil, garlic, milk alternatives, and foods with omega-3 fatty acids (found in nuts and seeds).

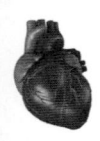

5. Avoid dairy products and eggs (contain cholesterol).

6. Keep your salt intake low (the body needs about 1 gram a day found mostly in foods 'as grown').

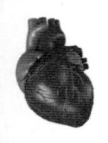

Excessive salt in the diet increases water retention, which increases blood volume, which raises blood pressure. Mostly highly processed and pre-packaged foods contain an incredible amount of salt and can quickly aggravate hypertension.
*Dr Peter N. Landless*

# 7. Have a regular exercise programme.

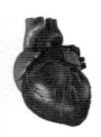

## A short walk
- 5-10 minutes, three times daily
- lowers apolipoprotein II (an LDL) 0.01 grams
- raises apolipoprotein I (an HDL)

## An intermediate walk
- 10-15 minutes, twice a day
- lowers apolipoprotein II 0.025 grams
- raises apolipoprotein I

## A long walk
- 20-40 minutes daily
- lowers apolipoprotein II 0.05 grams
- raises apolipoprotein I

8. Do not smoke, and, as far as possible, avoid the side-stream smoke of others.

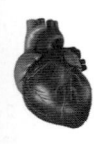

9. Avoid alcohol (the same protective effect can be gained from red-skinned fruits and vegetables, and in any case the amount of alcohol said to protect the heart will damage the brain and the liver).

# 10. Learn a good relaxation technique.

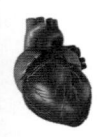

## The heart health risk test

For your score: Add up the numbers in each category that most nearly describes you.

Total_____

**Key to score:**
4-9 very remote
10-15 below average
16-20 average
21-25 moderate
26-30 dangerous
31-35 urgent danger, reduce score!
Other conditions, such as stress, high blood pressure and increased blood cholesterol detract from heart health and should be evaluated by your physician.

| Heredity | 1 No known history of heart disease | 2 One relative with heart disease over 60 years | 3 Two relatives with heart disease over 60 years | 4 One relative with heart disease under 60 years | 6 Two relatives with heart disease under 60 years |
|---|---|---|---|---|---|
| Exercise | 1 Intensive exercise, work and recreation | 2 Moderate exercise, work and recreation | 3 Sedentary work and intensive recreational exercise | 5 Sedentary work and moderate recreational exercise | 6 Sedentary work and light recreational exercise |
| Age | 1 10-20 | 2 21-30 | 3 31-40 | 4 41-50 | 6 51-65 |
| Load! (weight) | 0 More than 2.5kg below standard weight | 1 +/- 2.5kg standard weight | 2 2.5-10kg overweight | 4 10-15kg overweight | 6 15-22.5kg overweight |
| Tobacco | 0 Non-user | 1 Cigar or pipe | 2 10 cigarettes or less per day | 4 20 cigarettes or more per day | 6 30 cigarettes or more per day |
| Habits of eating fat | 1 0% No animal or solid fats | 2 10% Very little animal or solid fats | 3 20% Little animal or solid fats | 4 30% Much animal or solid fats | 5 40% Very much animal or solid fats |

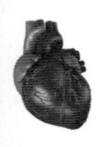

If you are really determined to join the **CORONARY CLUB**
1. Go to work every day, evenings, weekends and holidays.

2. Take work home with you and immerse yourself in your troubles and worries.

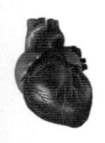

3. Show up early the next morning if you had a long night meeting.

4. Always opt for fast foods; never take healthful, relaxing meals.

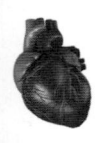

5. Look on any form of exercise as a waste of time.

6. Keep in contact with your work daily when on holiday or in hospital.

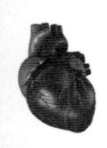

# 7. Do not delegate.

8. When travelling, work all day and drive all night to fill your day.

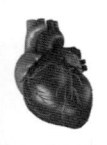

9. Accept all invitations to lunches, dinners and banquets, and join as many committees as possible.

10. Stay up all night writing sales reports, memos, and so on, (and while you are at it, an outline or detailed obituary!).

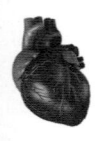

## Crisis point

If you are with someone who appears to have had a heart attack

1. Get help quickly for them.

2. Try to rouse them if they are unconscious.

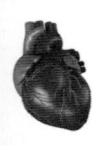

3. Check that their airways are clear.

4. Start mouth-to-mouth resuscitation and give them cardiac massage.

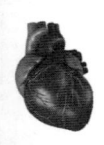

5. Give them an aspirin to chew if they are conscious.

## Blood flow may be restored by

- ♥ Medication.
- ♥ Angioplasty to dilate the blood vessel and/or introduce a stent to continue to dilate the artery.
- ♥ Surgery to 'replace' blood vessels or repair heart damage.

## However...

Despite the tremendous expense of bypass surgery and angioplasty, up to one half of bypass grafts become blocked again after only five to ten years, and one third to one half of angioplastied arteries close up after only four to six months, regardless of the method used.
*Dr Dean Ornish*

# PREVENTION is the CURE
*Dr Peter N. Landless*

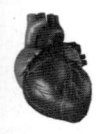

Meditation here
May think down hours to moments.
Here the heart
May give a useful lesson to the head,
And learning wiser grow without his books.
*William Cowper (1731-1800)*

Do your utmost to guard your heart, for out of it comes life.
*Walter Hilton*

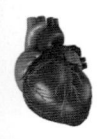

*'Let not your heart be troubled,'* said Jesus. *'Ye believe in God, believe also in me. In my Father's house are many mansions.... And if I go and prepare a place for you, I will come again...'*
John 14:1-3

*'Peace I leave with you,'* said Jesus, *'my peace I give unto you: not as the world giveth, give I unto you. Let not your heart be troubled, neither let it be afraid.'*
John 14:27

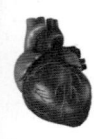

*In his heart a man plans his course, but the LORD determines his steps.*
*We plan the way we want to live, but only God makes us able to live it.*
Proverbs 16:9, NIV, MGE

*Jesus said, 'I will see you again, and your heart shall rejoice, and your joy no man taketh from you.'*
John 16:22

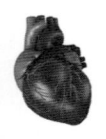

*Do you not know that your body is a temple of the Holy Spirit, who is in you, whom you have received from God? You are not your own; you were bought at a price. Therefore honour God with your body.*
1 Corinthians 6:19, 20, NIV